300 Questions and Answers in Anatomy and Physiology for Veterinary Nurses

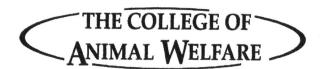

THE COLLEGE OF
ANIMAL WELFARE

Senior commissioning editor: Mary Seager
Editorial assistant: Caroline Savage
Production controller. Anthony Read
Desk editor: Angela Davies
Cover designer: Helen Brockway

300 Questions and Answers in Anatomy and Physiology for Veterinary Nurses

The College of Animal Welfare

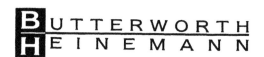

OXFORD   AUCKLAND   BOSTON
JOHANNESBURG   MELBOURNE   NEW DELHI

Butterworth-Heinemann
Linacre House, Jordan Hill, Oxford OX2 8DP
225 Wildwood Avenue, Woburn, MA 01801-2041
A division of Reed Educational and Professional Publishing Ltd

$\mathcal{R}$ A member of the Reed Elsevier plc group

First published 2000

British Library Cataloguing in Publication Data
300 questions and answers in anatomy and physiology. –
 (Veterinary nursing)
 1. Veterinary anatomy – Examinations, questions, etc.
 2. Veterinary physiology – Examinations, questions, etc.
 I. College of Animal Welfare   II. Three hundred questions and
answers in anatomy and physiology for veterinary nurses
 III. Anatomy and physiology for veterinary nurses
 636'.0892'0076

ISBN 0 7506 4695 0

Typeset by Keyword Typesetting Services, Wallington

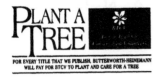

Contents

Acknowledgements   vi

Introduction   vii

Questions   1

Answers   79

Acknowledgements

The College is most grateful for the help of the following colleagues in the preparation of this book:

B. Cooper
B. Drysdale
D. Gould
J. Hargreaves
L. Tartaglia
A. Thomas
M. O'Reilly

Introduction

How the book is organized

This book of anatomy and physiology questions has been produced in response to further requests for more multiple choice questions.

It contains 300 questions covering anatomy and physiology. After the questions is a list of correct answers.

How to use the book

Do your revision first, then select a range of question numbers at random. Do this without looking at the questions in advance. You should be able to complete and finish one multiple choice question per minute, allowing time for a thorough read of the question and the options before selecting the correct answer.

Questions

1) *Which ONE of the following is a function of the periosteum?*

   a) To give attachment to tendons
   b) To supply nourishment to the bone
   c) To increase bone circumference
   d) To increase bone length

2) *A constituent of blood that is rich in antibodies is:*

   a) thromboplastin
   b) gamma-globulin
   c) leucocytes
   d) thrombocytes (platelets)

3) *Which ONE of the following is NOT a function of the blood?*

a) To provide materials for the manufacture of glandular secretions
b) To regulate body temperature
c) To cushion the brain and spinal cord
d) To arrest haemorrhage through clotting

4) *The interior of the heart is lined with:*

a) pericardium
b) endocardium
c) myometrium
d) endomysium

5) *The blood vessels which communicate with the left atrium of the heart are called:*

a) the pulmonary arteries
b) the coronary veins
c) the venae cavae
d) the pulmonary veins

6) *The sino-atrial node (pacemaker of the heart) is situated in the:*

a) wall of the right atrium
b) atrioventricular bundle (bundle of His)
c) atrioventricular node
d) wall of the right ventricle

7) *The function of the lymphatic capillaries is to carry:*

   a) food and oxygen from the bloodstream
   b) waste products from the cells to the bloodstream
   c) tissue fluid from the interstitial spaces to the lymphatic vessels
   d) intracellular fluid from the cells to the bloodstream

8) *Absorption of food occurs mainly from the:*

   a) stomach
   b) duodenum
   c) jejunum
   d) colon

9) *Haemopoiesis is:*

   a) destruction of red blood cells
   b) formation of antibodies in the blood
   c) process of blood clotting
   d) production of red blood cells

10) *Where is the ovum MOST likely to become fertilised?*

   a) Ovary
   b) Uterine tube (Fallopian tube)
   c) Uterine horn
   d) Uterine body

11) *The function of the prostate gland is to:*
   a) produce spermatazoa
   b) secrete testosterone
   c) secrete androgens
   d) secrete lubricant for spermatazoa

12) *Which ONE of the following produces spermatazoa?*
   a) Epididymis
   b) Interstitial cells of the testis
   c) Seminal vesicle
   d) Seminiferous tubules

13) *Trypsin is formed in the:*
   a) duodenum
   b) exocrine part of the pancreas
   c) islets of Langerhans
   d) stomach

14) *A catabolic reaction is:*
   a) the breakdown of starch to glucose with the
      liberation of energy
   b) where starch is broken down to glucose and where
      energy is necessary to bring it about
   c) the build up of starch from glucose with the
      liberation of energy
   d) the build up of starch from glucose and where
      energy is necessary to bring it about

15) *The dental formula of the kitten is:*

    a) I $\frac{3}{3}$ c $\frac{1}{1}$ pm $\frac{3}{3}$ m $\frac{0}{0}$ = 28

    b) I $\frac{3}{3}$ c $\frac{1}{1}$ pm $\frac{3}{2}$ m $\frac{1}{1}$ = 30

    c) I $\frac{3}{3}$ c $\frac{1}{1}$ pm $\frac{3}{3}$ m $\frac{1}{1}$ = 30

    d) I $\frac{3}{3}$ c $\frac{1}{1}$ pm $\frac{3}{2}$ m $\frac{0}{0}$ = 26

16) *Contraction of the quadriceps muscle produces:*

    a) extension of the hock
    b) extension of the stifle
    c) flexion of the hock
    d) flexion of the stifle

17) *The oestrous cycle of the bitch is divided into 4 stages. In order these are:*

    a) pro oestrus, anoestrus, metoestrus, oestrus
    b) oestrus, anoestrus, metoestrus, pro oestrus
    c) pro oestrus, metoestrus, oestrus, anoestrus
    d) pro oestrus, oestrus, metoestrus, anoestrus

18) *Intramembranous ossification is where:*

   a) the femur develops from a hyaline cartilage model
   b) the femur develops from primitive connective tissue
   c) the frontal bone develops from primitive connective tissue
   d) the parietal bone develops from transitional epithelial tissue

19) *The afferent lymphatic vessels:*

   a) take lymph to the lymph nodes, enter all over its surface and all are narrower in diameter than the corresponding efferent ones
   b) take lymph away from the lymph node, leaving at the hilus and are narrower in diameter than the corresponding efferent ones
   c) take lymph to the lymph node, enter at the hilus and are wider in diameter than the corresponding efferent ones
   d) take lymph away from the lymph node leaving at the hilus and are wider in diameter than the corresponding efferent ones

20) *The allantoic cavity is contained by cells originating from:*

   a) the endoderm
   b) the ectoderm
   c) the mesoderm
   d) the periderm

21) *Interstitial fluid is:*
   a) the fluid filling the spaces between cells
   b) the fluid inside cells
   c) only found in oedema
   d) 60% of body weight

22) *An animal dehydrated up to 5% of its weight loss will show:*
   a) inelastic skin
   b) dry mouth
   c) inelastic skin and dry mouth
   d) no clinical signs

23) *Renin is released from:*
   a) the kidney
   b) the pituitary
   c) the liver
   d) the adrenals

24) *Energy to run the cell's various activities is the result of cell respiration, which occurs in the:*
   a) ribosomes
   b) mitochondria
   c) Golgi bodies
   d) endoplasmic reticulum

25) *Which ONE of the following is located in the pelvic bone?*

   a) Foramen magnum
   b) Obturator foramen
   c) Supratrochlear foramen
   d) Intraorbital foramen

26) *A tendon connects:*

   a) bone to bone
   b) muscle to muscle
   c) muscle to bone
   d) ligament to bone

27) *The bladder is lined with:*

   a) smooth muscle
   b) elastic connective tissue
   c) transitional epithelium
   d) serous membrane

28) *The muscle that opens the jaw is the:*

   a) buccinator
   b) masseter
   c) digastricus
   d) temporalis

29) *The muscle that MOST completely covers the disto-*
lateral surface of the femur is the:

    a) gastrocnemius
    b) biceps femoris
    c) adductor
    d) semitendinosus

30) *In the cell, the organelle responsible for storage of*
digestive enzymes is:

    a) the lysosome
    b) the Golgi apparatus
    c) the endoplasmic reticulum
    d) the mitochondria

31) *How many sternebrae are there in the dog?*

    a) 8
    b) 9
    c) 10
    d) 11

32) *The layers of the epidermis are, in order from most superficial:*
   a) stratum germinativum, stratum granulosum, stratum lucidum, stratum corneum
   b) stratum lucidum, stratum corneum, stratum granulosum, stratum germinativum
   c) stratum corneum, stratum lucidum, stratum granulosum, stratum germinativum
   d) stratum granulosum, stratum germinativum, stratum lucidum, stratum corneum

33) *Internal respiration is the transfer of gases between:*
   a) the blood and body cells
   b) the environment and the lungs
   c) the environment and the lungs and the body cells
   d) the bronchi and the blood

34) *Inspiration is inhibited by:*
   a) blood CO_2 levels
   b) carbonic acid levels
   c) diaphragmatic contraction
   d) lung distension

35) *The cells that detect carbonic acid levels are situated in the:*
   a) carotid arteries and aorta
   b) carotid arteries
   c) aorta
   d) venae cavae

36) *Which ONE of the following is not a polymorphonuclear leucocyte?*

    a) Granulocyte
    b) Neutrophil
    c) Basophil
    d) Monocyte

37) *Three of the following vessels carry deoxygenated blood. Which ONE does NOT?*

    a) Pulmonary artery
    b) Pulmonary vein
    c) Coronary vein
    d) Portal vein

38) *Which ONE of the following is NOT a function of the spleen?*

    a) The manufacture of red blood cells
    b) The manufacture of white blood cells
    c) The breakdown of red blood cells
    d) The manufacture of antibodies

39) *Erythrocytes are destroyed in:*

    a) the pancreas
    b) the kidney
    c) the liver
    d) the bowel

40) *The outer layer of blood vessels is the:*
    a) tunica adventitia
    b) tunica media
    c) tunica intima
    d) squamous epithelial cells

41) *Which part of the myocardium is the thickest?*
    a) Right atrium
    b) Right ventricle
    c) Left atrium
    d) Left ventricle

42) *Heart muscle contraction is known as:*
    a) systole
    b) diastole
    c) emptying
    d) filling

43) *Which ONE of the following is not a superficial lymph node?*
    a) Inguinal
    b) Mesenteric
    c) Popliteal
    d) Axillary

44) *An isometric contraction:*

   a) moves a limb
   b) shortens a muscle
   c) tenses a muscle
   d) extends a limb

45) *The pectoral muscle is formed from:*

   a) striated muscle fibres
   b) unstriated muscle fibres
   c) smooth muscle fibres
   d) involuntary muscle fibres

46) *Which ONE of the following does NOT form part of the Achilles tendon?*

   a) Quadriceps femoris
   b) Semitendinosus
   c) Biceps femoris
   d) Gastrocnemius

47) *Which ONE of the following structures does NOT pass through the aortic hiatus?*

   a) Aorta
   b) Vagal nerve trunk
   c) Azygos vein
   d) Thoracic duct

48) *The muscles lying dorsally to the transverse processes of the vertebra are:*

   a) crura
   b) intercostal
   c) hypaxial
   d) epaxial

49) *The main muscle of respiration is the diaphragm. Where is it located?*

   a) Between the thorax and the abdomen
   b) Between the ribs
   c) At the thoracic inlet
   d) Cranial to the heart

50) *The three main muscle types are:*

   a) striped, skeletal and visceral
   b) smooth, unstriped and visceral
   c) striated, smooth and cardiac
   d) striped, skeletal and heart

51) *A hip adductor is found on which side of the femur?*

   a) Cranial
   b) Caudal
   c) Lateral
   d) Medial

52) *The muscle that flexes the stifle and extends the hock is the:*

   a) gastrocnemius
   b) biceps brachii
   c) triceps brachii
   d) sartorius

53) *Which muscle inserts on the olecranon?*

   a) Triceps brachii
   b) Biceps brachii
   c) Brachialis
   d) Teres major

54) *Which ONE of the following is not a function of the skin?*

   a) Protection
   b) Secretes pheromones
   c) Excretes waste products
   d) Vitamin A production

55) *Meibomian glands are present in the:*

   a) ear
   b) eyelid
   c) body skin
   d) tail gland

56) *Horny nail growth takes place at the:*

   a) claw sole
   b) claw fold
   c) coronary band
   d) the quick

57) *The epidermis is made up of:*

   a) ciliated columnar epithelium
   b) stratified squamous epithelium
   c) transitional epithelium
   d) simple squamous epithelium

58) *Milk does NOT contain:*

   a) protein
   b) lactose
   c) vitamin B
   d) vitamin D

59) *Which ONE of the following is NOT a function of the integument?*

   a) Secretion and excretion
   b) Sensation
   c) Synthesis of vitamin E
   d) Temperature regulation

60) *The arrector pili muscles are attached to the:*

   a) guard hairs
   b) hair beds
   c) hair clusters
   d) wool hairs

61) *The oil glands of the skin are the:*

   a) anal glands
   b) mammary glands
   c) sebaceous glands
   d) sudoriferous glands

62) *Chromosomes are made up of:*

   a) chromic fibres
   b) cilia
   c) chromatin fibres
   d) collagen fibres

63) *Genes that can occupy the same gene locus are called:*

   a) similar
   b) genetic
   c) chromosomal
   d) allelomorphic

64) *When alleles are identical they are called:*

a) homozygous
b) heterozygous
c) autosomal
d) homologous

65) *The outward appearance of an animal is its:*

a) genotype
b) phenotype
c) autosomal
d) homologous

66) *Which one of the following stages of mitosis is in the correct order?*

a) Interphase, prophase, anaphase, metaphase, telophase
b) Interphase, prophase, metaphase, telophase, anaphase
c) Interphase, prophase, metaphase, anaphase, telophase
d) Interphase, prophase, telophase, anaphase, metaphase

67) *If a black Labrador (Bb) is mated with a chocolate Labrador (bb), what percentage of the litter will be black?*

a) 100%
b) 50%
c) 25%
d) 0%

68) *The gene for the tortoiseshell coat colour in cats is:*

a) mutation
b) epistatic
c) sex limiting
d) sex linked

69) *Which ONE of the following is in the correct sequence?*

a) Ingestion, digestion, absorption, assimilation
b) Digestion, absorption, assimilation, ingestion
c) Digestion, ingestion, assimilation, absorption
d) Ingestion, assimilation, digestion, absorption

70) *Bile is:*

a) very acidic
b) slightly acidic
c) neutral
d) alkaline

71) *Deamination is:*

   a) the conversion of glucose to glycogen
   b) the conversion of glycogen to glucose
   c) the breakdown of amino acids
   d) the conversion of amino acids

72) *Trypsin is an enzyme that:*

   a) is produced in the stomach
   b) requires an alkaline environment
   c) digests carbohydrates
   d) is the precursor of trypsinogen

73) *Oxyntic cells produce:*

   a) hydrochloric acid
   b) pepsinogen
   c) renin
   d) mucus

74) *Glycerol is the breakdown product of:*

   a) protein
   b) carbohydrates
   c) fats
   d) minerals

75) *The cells that detect oxygen levels in the blood are located in:*

   a) the aorta
   b) the carotid arteries
   c) the brain stem
   d) the aorta and the carotid arteries

76) *What is the term used to describe the effect which stops the lungs overinflating?*

   a) The Hering-Bruer effect
   b) The Kelsey effect
   c) The medulla oblongata
   d) The rideal effect

77) *The nucleus of a cell is an essential part of all body cells except for:*

   a) liver cells
   b) immature red blood cells
   c) kidney cells
   d) mature red blood cells

78) *The golden brown pigment found in cells which are connected with haemoglobin breakdown is called:*

   a) melanin
   b) haemosiderin
   c) mitochondria
   d) cytoplasm

79) *Oxytocin and vasopressin are released from the:*

a) adrenal glands
b) anterior pituitary
c) hypothalamus
d) posterior pituitary

80) *Which ONE of the following statements is the most accurate? The lacrimal gland:*

a) is ventral to the eyeball
b) secretes fluid that drains from the orbital region into the nasal vestibule
c) secretes fluid that enters the anterior chamber of the eye
d) secretes fluid that enters the conjunctival sac through the caudal surface of the third eyelid

81) *The uveal tract consists of:*

a) choroid, iris and retina
b) choroid, ciliary body and iris
c) choroid, ciliary body and lens
d) choroid, ciliary body and retina

82) *Glucagon is secreted by which type of pancreatic islet cell?*

a) Alpha cells
b) Beta cells
c) Gamma cells
d) Delta cells

83) *Rotary motion of the head is detected by which sensory structure?*

   a) Cochlea
   b) Organ of Corti
   c) Semicircular canal
   d) Vestibule

84) *Which ONE of these statement is TRUE?*

   a) Thyroid hormone increases resorption of calcium from bone
   b) Thyroid hormone raises the metabolic rate of the body
   c) Thyroid hormone reduces the metabolic rate of the body
   d) Thyroid hormone reduces the resorption of calcium and phosphorous in the kidney

85) *Which cardiac chamber receives blood from the systemic veins?*

   a) Right ventricle
   b) Right atrium
   c) Left atrium
   d) Left ventricle

86) *Which vessel normally carries blood with a high level of carbon dioxide?*

a) Carotid artery
b) Pulmonary vein
c) Umbilical vein
d) Vena cava

87) *The average life span of a circulating erythrocyte in mammalian blood is approximately:*

a) 90 days
b) 100 days
c) 110 days
d) 120 days

88) *The coronary arteries are branches of the:*

a) aorta
b) left atrium
c) pulmonary trunk
d) right atrium

89) *The hepatic portal system carries:*

a) blood from the heart to the liver via the aorta
b) blood from the intestines to the liver capillaries
c) lymph from the intestines to the heart via the thoracic duct
d) lymph from the lacteals to the hepatic vein

90) *White blood cells are divided into granulocytes and agranulocytes. Which cell is an agranulocyte?*

   a) Monocyte
   b) Neutrophil
   c) Eosinophil
   d) Basophil

91) *The name of the valve that separates the left atrium and left ventricle in the heart is the:*

   a) tricuspid valve
   b) mitral valve
   c) pulmonic valve
   d) aortic valve

92) *Which muscle type is under voluntary control?*

   a) Smooth muscle
   b) Skeletal muscle
   c) Uterine muscle
   d) Cardiac muscle

93) *A motor unit is made up of:*

   a) a neuron and tendon
   b) a muscle fibre and tendon
   c) a neuron and muscle fibre
   d) a muscle fibre and bone

94) *Epaxial muscles of the vertebrae lie* _____ *to the transverse processes?*

   a) Dorsal
   b) Ventral
   c) Medial
   d) Lateral

95) *The linea alba is the area where which muscles come together?*

   a) Epaxial muscles
   b) Quadriceps femoris muscles
   c) Thoracic muscles
   d) Abdominal muscles

96) *The triceps muscle of the forelimb:*

   a) extends the elbow
   b) flexes the elbow
   c) extends the shoulder
   d) flexes the shoulder

97) *The biceps muscle of the forelimb:*

   a) extends the elbow
   b) flexes the elbow
   c) extends the shoulder
   d) flexes the shoulder

98) *Which ONE of the following is NOT part of the gluteal group of muscles?*

    a) Minimus
    b) Micromus
    c) Medius
    d) Maximus

99) *The gastrocnemius muscle:*

    a) extends the stifle
    b) flexes the stifle
    c) extends the tarsus
    d) flexes the tarsus

100) *The supra spinatus muscle:*

    a) flexes the shoulder joint
    b) extends the shoulder joint
    c) flexes the elbow joint
    d) extends the elbow joint

101) *In young growing animals, growth in length of long bones occurs at the:*

    a) epithelium
    b) periosteum
    c) diaphysis
    d) epiphyseal plate

102) *The term phagocytosis is used to describe the process whereby cells:*

a) manufacture protein
b) manufacture carbohydrates
c) eliminate waste products
d) destroy invading bacteria and debris

103) *Which is the hardest substance in the animal body?*

a) cartilage
b) bone
c) dentine
d) enamel

104) *Which two structures make up the joint capsule?*

a) synovial membrane and hyaline cartilage
b) synovial membrane and fibrous membrane
c) fibrous membrane and hyaline cartilage
d) fibrous membrane and capsular ligament

105) *The calcaneus is found:*

a) in the hock
b) in the stifle
c) in the elbow
d) in the carpus

106) *Hyaline cartilage is found in:*

   a) intervertebral discs
   b) the mandibular symphysis
   c) fibrocartilaginous joints
   d) synovial joints

107) *An intra-articular meniscus:*

   a) is made of elastic cartilage
   b) is found in the temporo-mandibular joint
   c) helps to stabilise a joint
   d) replaces the articular cartilage within a joint

108) *Which ONE of the following types of gland secretes directly into the bloodstream?*

   a) Mucous
   b) Simple
   c) Compound
   d) Endocrine

109) *Which ONE of the following is an example of an exocrine gland?*

   a) Adrenal
   b) Salivary
   c) Pituitary
   d) Ovary

110) *Body tissues are all classified into four types:*

    a) epithelial, glandular, connective, bone
    b) nervous, squamous, nervous, skeletal
    c) epithelial, glandular, nervous, skeletal
    d) epithelial, connective, muscular, nervous

111) *The predominant type of connective tissue in tendons and ligaments is:*

    a) areolar connective tissue
    b) dense fibrous connective tissue
    c) elastic connective tissue
    d) fibrocartilage

112) *A muscle that increases the angle between two bones is known as:*

    a) an abductor
    b) an adductor
    c) an extensor
    d) a flexor

113) *The femur is an example of a:*

    a) long bone
    b) short bone
    c) flat bone
    d) irregular bone

114) *The scapula is an example of a:*

   a) long bone
   b) short bone
   c) flat bone
   d) irregular bone

115) *The manubrium is found:*

   a) in the lower jaw
   b) in the pelvis
   c) between the two pelvic bones
   d) in the sternum

116) *During endochondral ossification, the primary centre of ossification develops:*

   a) in the epiphysis
   b) in the diaphysis
   c) at the epiphyseal plate
   d) in the growth cartilage

117) *Secondary centres of ossification then develop:*

   a) in the epiphysis
   b) in the diaphysis
   c) at the epiphyseal plate
   d) in the growth cartilage

118) *Which ONE of the following bones is NOT part of the axial skeleton?*

 a) The mandible
 b) The sternebrae
 c) The sacrum
 d) The phalanges

119) *Which ONE of the following bones is NOT part of the appendicular skeleton?*

 a) The fibula
 b) The calcaneus
 c) The scapula
 d) The sacrum

120) *An example of a condylar joint is:*

 a) the hip
 b) the shoulder
 c) the elbow
 d) the carpus

121) *An example of a hinge joint is:*

 a) an intervertebral joint
 b) the stifle joint
 c) the hip joint
 d) the sacroiliac joint

122) *Simple cuboidal epithelium is found:*

    a) in the bronchi of the respiratory tract
    b) lining the kidney tubules
    c) lining body cavities
    d) in the small intestine

123) *Simple columnar epithelium is found:*

    a) in the bronchi of the respiratory tract
    b) lining the kidney tubules
    c) lining body cavities
    d) in the small intestine

124) *Simple squamous epithelium is found:*

    a) in the bronchi of the respiratory tract
    b) lining the kidney tubules
    c) lining body cavities
    d) in the small intestine

125) *The alveoil are lined with:*

    a) simple squamous epithelium
    b) ciliated mucous epithelium
    c) stratified squamous epithelium
    d) transitional epithelium

126) *The following are all types of connective tissue:*

   a) loose connective tissue, fibrous connective tissue, muscle, blood

   b) areolar tissue, adipose tissue, cartilage, nerve

   c) bone, cartilage, skin, blood

   d) cartilage, dense connective tissue, bone, blood

127) *Which ONE of the following muscle types has branching cells within its structure?*

   a) Skeletal muscle

   b) Striated muscle

   c) Smooth muscle

   d) Cardiac muscle

128) *Which ONE of the following muscle types is found in the wall of the intestine?*

   a) Skeletal muscle

   b) Striated muscle

   c) Smooth muscle

   d) Cardiac muscle

129) *Which ONE of the following is NOT a function of skin?*

   a) Temperature regulation

   b) Protection against micro-organisms

   c) Vitamin manufacture

   d) Antibody production

130) *Which ONE of the following breeds of dog does not moult?*

   a) The Standard poodle
   b) The Bichon Frise
   c) The Bedlington terrier
   d) All of the above

131) *Which ONE of the following structures is NOT associated with the hair follicles on the dorsum (back) of the normal dog?*

   a) Sebaceous gland
   b) Sweat gland
   c) Arrector pili muscle
   d) Wool hairs

132) *Inspired air consists of:*

   a) 29% nitrogen
   b) 79% nitrogen
   c) 89% nitrogen
   d) 21% nitrogen

133) *Which ONE of the following is least accurate?*

   a) Nitrogen is unchanged in expired air
   b) Oxygen levels in expired air are lower
   c) Water vapour is slightly higher in inspired air
   d) Carbon dioxide levels are lower in inspired air

134) *Which ONE of the following is least accurate?*

   a) The trachea is a permanently open tube
   b) The oesophagus lies above the trachea
   c) The trachea cartilages are open on the dorsal aspect
   d) The tracheal cartilages are open on the ventral aspect

135) *Which ONE of the following sequences is correct with regard to what happens when the trachea splits into two?*

   a) Trachea, bronchi, bronchioles, alveolar duct, alveolar sac
   b) Trachea, bronchi, bronchioles, alveolar sac, alveolar duct
   c) Trachea, bronchioles, bronchi, alveolar sac, alveolar duct
   d) Trachea, bronchioles, bronchi, alveolar duct, alveolar sac

136) *Which structure does NOT lie within the mediastinum?*

   a) Heart
   b) Oesophagus
   c) Trachea
   d) Lungs

137) *Which is NOT a feature of the larynx?*

   a) It produces sound
   b) It is shared by the digestive and respiratory tracts
   c) It plays a role in swallowing
   d) It forms the opening into the trachea

138) *Which ONE of the following would NOT cause a decreased respiratory rate?*

   a) Pyrexia
   b) Sleep
   c) Anaesthesia
   d) Inactivity

139) *The epithelium found lining the GI tract is known as:*

   a) Stratified squamous epithelium
   b) Simple columnar epithelium
   c) Ciliated columnar epithelium
   d) Simple squamous epithelium

140) *Which ONE of the following is NOT an exocrine gland?*

   a) Sebaceous gland
   b) Anal gland
   c) Salivary gland
   d) Thyroid gland

141) *Which ONE of the following is a type of connective tissue?*

   a) Fibrocartilage
   b) Compact bone
   c) Adipose tissue
   d) All of the above

142) *Which organ is NOT part of the upper urinary tract?*

   a) Bladder
   b) Kidney
   c) Urethra
   d) Ureter

143) *Which structure does NOT enter or leave the hilus of the kidney?*

   a) Blood vessels
   b) Nerves
   c) Renal pelvis
   d) Uterus

144) *The outer portion of the kidney is:*

   a) medulla
   b) hilus
   c) renal pelvis
   d) cortex

145) *Which part of the nephron is NOT found in the cortex of the kidney?*

    a) Glomerulus

    b) Loop of Henle

    c) PCT

    d) DCT

146) *Blood enters the glomerulus via:*

    a) afferent arteriole

    b) efferent arteriole

    c) renal artery

    d) afferent venule

147) *Which part of the nephron is found in the medulla of the kidney?*

    a) PCT

    b) DCT

    c) Bowman's capsule

    d) Loop of Henle

148) *Which hormone is NOT produced by the kidney?*

    a) Erythropoietin

    b) Renin

    c) Anti-diuretic hormone

    d) Fhyroxine

149) *Which part of the nephron acts as a filter of plasma?*

   a) PCT
   b) Glomerulus
   c) DCT
   d) Loop of Henle

150) *Which hormone is responsible for increasing reabsorption of sodium?*

   a) Aldosterone
   b) Vitamin D
   c) Renin
   d) Erythropoietin

151) *Which ONE of the following is NOT a function of oestrogen?*

   a) Development of mammary glands
   b) Thickening of endometrium
   c) Maintains pregnancy
   d) Increases receptiveness during oestrus

152) *Which muscles help contribute to the tie ?*

   a) Vaginal
   b) Cervix
   c) Vulval
   d) Vestibular

153) *Which ONE of the following is NOT a sign of pro-oestrus?*

   a) Swollen vulva
   b) Behaviour changes
   c) Clear discharge
   d) Slightly increased receptiveness to the male

154) *The uterus is supported in the abdomen by a fold of peritoneum called the:*

   a) broad ligament
   b) round ligament
   c) myometrium
   d) ovarian ligament

155) *The inner layer of the uterus is the:*

   a) myometrium
   b) mycometrium
   c) endometrium
   d) endoderm

156) *The hormone responsible for the maintenance of pregnancy in the bitch is:*

   a) FSH: follicle stimulating hormone
   b) LH: luteinising hormone
   c) oestradiol
   d) progesterone

157) *The layer of peritoneum covering the testes is known as:*

   a) tunica externa
   b) tunica vasculosa
   c) tunica vaginalis
   d) tunica spermatica

158) *The sertoli cells produce:*

   a) oestrogen
   b) testosterone
   c) progesterone
   d) sperm

159) *Testosterone is NOT responsible for:*

   a) male behaviour
   b) development of the prostate
   c) descent of the testes
   d) nutrition for spermatozoa

160) *Sperm leaves the epididymis in:*

   a) afferent ducts
   b) efferent ducts
   c) vas deferens
   d) seminiferous tubules

161) *The glans-penis consists of the:*

    a) corpus spongiosum
    b) corpus cavernosum
    c) erectile tissue
    d) none of the above

162) *Which ONE of the following is the LEAST accurate?*

    a) The dog's penis points cranially
    b) The dog's scrotum lies between the hind limbs
    c) The dog's prostate lies near to the os-penis
    d) The dog's os-penis lies dorsal to the urethra

163) *Another name for the interstitial cells of the testis is:*

    a) accessory cells
    b) Leydig cells
    c) seminiferous cells
    d) Sertoli cells

164) *Spermatogenesis takes place in the:*

    a) epididymis
    b) seminal vesicles
    c) seminiferous tubules
    d) vas deferens

165) *Which ONE of the following has two uteri?*

   a) Snake
   b) Guinea pig
   c) Tortoise
   d) Rabbit

166) *Which ONE of the following is not a function of the spleen?*

   a) Phagocytosis
   b) Storage of red blood cells
   c) Absorption of nutrients
   d) Destruction of red blood cells

167) *Which ONE is not an example of lymphoid tissue?*

   a) Tonsils
   b) Thymus
   c) Spleen
   d) Villus

168) *A lacteal is what?*

   a) Lymphatic capillary
   b) Lymphatic duct
   c) Lymphatic vessel
   d) Lymph node

169) *Which ONE of the following structures produces lymphocytes?*

   a) Lymph nodes
   b) Spleen
   c) Thymus
   d) All of the above

170) *What do lymphocytes produce?*

   a) Tissue fluid
   b) Lymph
   c) Antibodies
   d) Antigens

171) *Where is the thymus found?*

   a) Throat
   b) Abdomen
   c) Thorax
   d) Stomach

172) *The portion of the lymphatic duct in the abdomen is called:*

   a) thoracic duct
   b) abdominal duct
   c) afferent duct
   d) cysterna chyli

173) *Which ONE of the following lymph nodes could be palpated in the groin of the dog?*

   a) Superficial inguinal
   b) Axillary
   c) Prescapular
   d) Popliteal

174) *Which ONE of the following is NOT usually indicative of hypothyroidism?*

   a) Hypothermia
   b) Weight loss
   c) Reduced appetite
   d) Low exercise tolerance

175) *Which ONE of the following statements is true?*

   a) Parathormone reduces calcium resorption in the kidney
   b) Parathormone in reduced quantities may cause hyperthyroidism
   c) Parathormone decreases calcium reabsorption from the bone
   d) Parathormone increases calcium absorption from the gut

176) *Hormones produced by this gland regulate metabolism, water balance and some sex steroids. It is the:*

   a) thyroid
   b) ovaries
   c) adrenal cortex
   d) adrenal medulla

177) *The adrenal medulla secretes:*

   a) adrenaline
   b) epinephrine
   c) norepinephrine
   d) all of the above

178) *Anti-diuretic hormone is produced by:*

   a) anterior pituitary gland
   b) posterior pituitary gland
   c) kidney
   d) adrenal glands

179) *Which ONE of the following hormones is NOT produced by the anterior pituitary gland?*

   a) Relaxin
   b) Adrenocorticotrophic hormone
   c) Follicle stimulating hormone
   d) Interstitial cell stimulating hormone

180) *Which TWO hormones are produced by the pituitary gland and have a direct effect on the ovary?*

   a) Follicle–stimulating hormone and progesterone
   b) Progesterone and luteinising hormone
   c) Follicle–stimulating hormone and luteinising hormone
   d) Progesterone and oestrogen

181) *Which ONE of the salivary glands secretes ptyalin (amylase)?*

   a) Parotid
   b) Submandibular
   c) Sublingual
   d) Zygomatic

182) *Trypsin digests:*

   a) complex carbohydrates
   b) proteins
   c) sucrose
   d) unsaturated fatty acids

183) *The stomach of the dog produces hydrochloric acid, mucus and:*

   a) amylase
   b) bile salts
   c) pepsin
   d) trypsin

184) *The stomach of the dog is divided into three parts, which from the entrance of the oesophagus are termed:*

a) cardia, fundus and pylorus
b) fundus, cardia and pylorus
c) fundus, pylorus and cardia
d) pylorus, cardia and fundus

185) *The major site for water absorption in the gut is the:*

a) colon
b) rectum
c) small intestine
d) stomach

186) *The function of ptyalin is:*

a) to maintain an alkaline pH
b) to start the digestion of carbohydrate
c) to stimulate the release of mucus by the gland
d) to stimulate the secretion of bicarbonate

187) *Which ONE of the following statements is INCORRECT?*

a) The pH of pancreatic juice is acidic
b) The wall of the small intestine contains smooth muscle
c) Bile is produced in the liver
d) Bile enters the small intestine at the duodenum

188) *The exocrine pancreas assists in the process of digestion by producing:*

   a) amylase, bile acids, bile salts and trypsin
   b) amylase, bile acids, pepsin and bicarbonate ions
   c) amylase, lipase, trypsin and bicarbonate ions
   d) amylase, lipase, trypsin and gastrin

189) *The enzyme pepsin is produced in the:*

   a) intestinal juice and breaks down carbohydrate
   b) pancreatic juice and breaks down protein
   c) stomach and breaks down carbohydrate
   d) stomach and breaks down protein

190) *Fats that are digested and absorbed into lacteals are then carried almost directly into the:*

   a) cisterna chyli
   b) hepatic vein
   c) portal vein
   d) right azygos vein

191) *Which ONE of the following statements is INCORRECT?*

   a) Bile contains enzymes to aid fat digestion
   b) Bile contains pigments which are waste products of haemoglobin breakdown
   c) Bile is produced in the liver
   d) Bile contains bicarbonate and electrolytes

192) *Chyme is:*

   a) the mix of food, mucus and gastric secretions produced in the stomach
   b) the milky fluid contained within the thoracic duct
   c) the enzyme used to break down fats
   d) the exocrine secretion produced by the pancreas

193) *The small intestine is divided into three sections. In which order does food pass through them?*

   a) Duodenum, ileum, jejunum
   b) Jejunum, ileum, duodenum
   c) Ileum, duodenum, jejunum
   d) Duodenum, jejunum, ileum

194) *In which part of the intestinal tract would you find villi?*

   a) Stomach
   b) Small intestine
   c) Rectum
   d) Colon

195) *Which ONE of the following is the correct formulae for the dog's permanent teeth?*

   a) I 3/3 C 1/1 PM 3/3 M 2/3
   b) I 3/3 C 1/1 PM 3/3 M 3/2
   c) I 3/3 C 1/1 PM 4/4 M 3/2
   d) I 3/3 C 1/1 PM 4/4 M 2/3

196) *In the dog the carnassial tooth is:*

    a) M1 lower jaw
    b) PM3 upper jaw
    c) PM4 upper jaw
    d) M1 upper jaw

197) *Vessels returning blood to the heart are generally:*

    a) capillaries
    b) veins
    c) arteries
    d) arterioles

198) *The vessels which transport blood to the capillaries are the:*

    a) venules
    b) veins
    c) arteries
    d) arterioles

199) *Erythrocytes are:*

    a) white blood cells
    b) red blood cells
    c) platelets
    d) both a + b

200) *A thrombocyte is:*

   a) a red blood cell
   b) a white blood cell
   c) a blood platelet
   d) a blood parasite

201) *The normal pulse rate for a dog is:*

   a) 60–180 bpm
   b) 60–120 bpm
   c) 70–140 bpm
   d) 80–160 bpm

202) *Which blood vessels contain valves?*

   a) Arteries
   b) Veins
   c) Arterioles
   d) Both a + c

203) *Which artery supplies the head with blood?*

   a) Anterior vena cava
   b) Posterior vena cava
   c) Hepatic artery
   d) Aorta

204)   *The right atrioventricular valve is also known as:*

a) the bicuspid valve
b) the mitral valve
c) the tricuspid valve
d) the pulmonary valve

205)   *Which blood vessel carries blood from the small intestine to the liver?*

a) Hepatic vein
b) Hepatic artery
c) Aorta
d) Hepatic portal vein

206)   *Which ONE of the following is INCORRECT?*

a) Blood leaving the left ventricle is oxygenated
b) Blood in the pulmonary vein is deoxygenated
c) Blood leaving the liver is deoxygenated
d) Blood entering the right atrium is deoxygenated

207)   *Oxygen forms approximately what percentage of normal inspired air?*

a) 20%
b) 40%
c) 60%
d) 80%

208) *Accommodation for near and far vision is accomplished by contraction or relaxation of the muscles in the:*

   a) ciliary body
   b) conjunctiva
   c) iris
   d) limbus

209) *The vitreous body of the canine eye:*

   a) is formed by the ciliary body
   b) is located within the posterior chamber of the eye
   c) is firmly attached to the caudal part of the eye
   d) forms the tapetum lucidum

210) *The tissue found lining the pleural cavity is:*

   a) simple squamous epithelium
   b) simple cuboidal epithelium
   c) simple columnar epithelium
   d) ciliated columnar epithelium

211) *The cell body of the sensory neuron within a simple reflex arc is placed:*

   a) in the dorsal horn
   b) in the ventral horn
   c) in the dorsal root ganglion
   d) in the ventral root ganglion

212) *The zygomatic arch is:*

  a) on the side of the skull
  b) attached to the pelvis
  c) the curve of the caudal border of the ribcage
  d) on the base of the skull

213) *An electron:*

  a) carries a positive charge
  b) carries a negative charge
  c) has an atomic weight of 1
  d) lies within the nucleus of the atom

214) *The nucleus of the atom is made up of:*

  a) protons and electrons
  b) electrons and neutrons
  c) protons and neutrons
  d) protons, neutrons and electrons

215) *Isotopes of an element have:*

  a) the same atomic number and the same atomic weight
  b) the same atomic number and different atomic weight
  c) the same atomic weight but a different atomic number
  d) different atomic number and weight from one another

216) *Which group of vertebrae have, on average, the longest dorsal spines?*

   a) Cervical
   b) Thoracic
   c) Lumbar
   d) Sacral

217) *The thoracic cavity is lined with a serous membrane called the:*

   a) peritoneum
   b) perineum
   c) pleura
   d) mediastinum

218) *The chemical used by the mitochondria within the cells as a means of storing energy is:*

   a) adenosine triphosphate
   b) phospholipid
   c) calcium phosphate
   d) mucopolysaccharide

219) *Which term means a decrease in the white blood cell count?*

   a) Lymphocytosis
   b) Leucocytosis
   c) Leucopaenia
   d) Anaemia

220) *Cornified stratified squamous epithelium is found:*

   a) on the skin surface
   b) lining the respiratory tract
   c) lining the major blood vessels
   d) on the surface of the eye

221) *If the Achilles tendon is torn, the animal loses most of its ability to:*

   a) extend the stifle
   b) extend the hip
   c) extend the hock
   d) flex the hock

222) *The patella is normally:*

   a) within the tendon of the gastrocnemius muscle
   b) attached to the medial meniscus of the stifle joint
   c) within the tendon of insertion of biceps femoris
   d) positioned proximal to the femoro-tibial joint space

223) *There are a number of foramina or hiati that pass through the diaphragm. Which of them passes through the central tendinous area?*

   a) The post-caval foramen
   b) The oesophageal hiatus
   c) The aortic hiatus
   d) The azygal foramen

224) *Within bone, the blood vessels are situated:*

  a) within the lacunae
  b) in the Haversian canals
  c) only within the marrow cavity
  d) Nowhere. Bone is avascular

225) *Which ONE of the following muscles is NOT a member of the hamstring group?*

  a) Semimembranosus
  b) Quadriceps femoris
  c) Semitendinosus
  d) Biceps femoris

226) *The main extensor of the shoulder is:*

  a) biceps brachii
  b) brachialis
  c) triceps brachii
  d) supraspinatus

227) *The inguinal ring is a hole in the aponeurosis of which abdominal muscle?*

  a) External abdominal oblique
  b) Internal abdominal oblique
  c) Tranversus abdominis
  d) Rectus abdominis

228) *How many pairs of mammary glands are MOST common in the bitch ?*

a) 3
b) 4
c) 5
d) 6

229) *Which type of joint movement decreases the angle between two bones?*

a) Abduction
b) Adduction
c) Extension
d) Flexion

230) *The second heart sound is produced by closure of which heart valves?*

a) Aortic and mitral
b) Mitral and pulmonary
c) Pulmonary and aortic
d) Pulmonary and tricuspid

231) *The first heart sound is produced by closure of which heart valves?*

a) Aortic and mitral
b) Mitral and pulmonary
c) Mitral and tricuspid
d) Pulmonary and aortic

232) *Inspiration of air into the lungs is produced by contraction of the:*

   a) Abdmominal oblique muscles
   b) Diaphragm
   c) Internal intercostal muscles
   d) Rectus abdominis muscles

233) *Which ONE of the following is not a function of the respiratory system?*

   a) Acid-base regulation
   b) Phonation
   c) Prehension
   d) Temperature regulation

234) *Oxygen and carbon dioxide are transferred between inspired air and blood in the lung by the process of:*

   a) flow down the pressure gradient
   b) diffusion
   c) ion pumping
   d) nitrogenation

235) *Which organ has endocrine functions and also produces many digestive enzymes?*

   a) Kidney
   b) Liver
   c) Pancreas
   d) Spleen

236) *Stimulation of the parasympathetic portion of the autonomic nervous system causes:*

   a) dilation of airways in the lung
   b) dilation of the pupil of the eye
   c) increased gastrointestinal function
   d) increased blood pressure

237) *Stimulation of the sympathetic portion of the autonomic nervous system causes all of the following except:*

   a) dilation of the pupil of the eye
   b) increased gastrointestinal function
   c) increased heart rate
   d) piloerection

238) *The part of the central nervous system that initiates conscious movements of the body is the:*

   a) brachial plexus
   b) brain stem
   c) cerebellum
   d) spinal cord

239) *Concerning neurons, which statement is least accurate?*

   a) They cannot replicate themselves
   b) They cannot regenerate damaged processes
   c) They contain no blood vessels
   d) They have a very high oxygen requirement

240) *Damage to which part of the nervous system is MOST likely to cause instant death in an animal?*

   a) Brachial plexus
   b) Brain stem
   c) Cerebellum
   d) Cerebrum

241) *Which structure is the MOST important direct link between the nervous and endocrine systems?*

   a) Hypothalamus
   b) Parathyroid gland
   c) Pituitary gland
   d) Thalamus

242) *Which hormone is produced by the anterior pituitary gland?*

   a) Antidiuretic hormone
   b) Calcitonin
   c) Luteinising hormone
   d) Oxytocin

243) *Which hormone is released by the posterior pituitary gland?*

   a) Adrenocorticotrophic hormone
   b) Calcitonin
   c) Luteinising hormone
   d) Oxytocin

244) *Which hormone is produced by the corpus luteum of the ovary?*

   a) Oestrogen
   b) Luteinising hormone
   c) Oxytocin
   d) Progesterone

245) *The hormone necessary for maintenance of pregnancy is:*

   a) oestrogen
   b) oxytocin
   c) progesterone
   d) prolactin

246) *Which hormone is produced by a developing follicle in the ovary?*

   a) Oestrogen
   b) Follicle-stimulating hormone
   c) Luteinising hormone
   d) Progesterone

247) *Which endocrine gland releases the hormone that causes milk letdown from the mammary gland?*

   a) Adrenal cortex
   b) Anterior pituitary gland
   c) Ovary
   d) Posterior pituitary gland

248) *Hormones of the adrenal medulla are released under the influence of:*

   a) adrenomedullotrophic hormone
   b) the parasympathetic nervous system
   c) the somatic nervous system
   d) the sympathetic nervous system

249) *The kidney helps control water balance in the body under the influence of:*

   a) adrenocorticotrophic hormone
   b) antidiuretic hormone
   c) calcitonin
   d) oxytocin

250) *In dogs, seminal fluid is produced by the:*

   a) prostate gland, seminal vesicles and bulbourethral glands
   b) prostate gland and seminal vesicles
   c) prostate gland
   d) seminal vesicles

251) *After spermatogenesis, spermatozoa are stored until ejaculation in the:*

   a) epididymis
   b) seminal vesicles
   c) seminiferous tubules
   d) vas deferens

252) *During which stage of the oestrous cycle do bitches allow dogs to copulate?*

a) Anoestrus
b) Dioestrus
c) Oestrus
d) Metoestrus

253) *Fertilisation of an ovum by a spermatozoon normally occurs in the:*

a) cervix
b) oviduct
c) uterus
d) vagina

254) *The process of capacitation of spermatozoa normally occurs in the:*

a) cervix
b) epididymis
c) oviduct
d) testes

255) *Milk letdown in the mammary gland is stimulated by:*

a) growth hormone
b) oxytocin
c) progesterone
d) prolactin

256) *Which anterior pituitary hormone stimulates spermatogenesis in males?*

a) Follicle-stimulating hormone
b) Growth hormone
c) Luteinising hormone
d) Prolactin

257) *Which hormone is responsible for the signs of heat in a female animal?*

a) Oestrogen
b) Follicle-stimulating hormone
c) Oxytocin
d) Progesterone

258) *Which ONE of the following statements concerning blood is TRUE?*

a) Contains cells and plasma
b) Is not important for CO_2 transport
c) Consists of cells and serum
d) Has no excretory function

259) *The major determinant of blood viscosity is the:*

a) specific gravity of plasma
b) plasma protein concentration
c) lipoprotein concentration
d) haematocrit

260) *Circulating blood volume is regulated primarily by control of:*

   a) total body water volume
   b) intracellular water volume
   c) systemic arterial blood pressure
   d) plasma protein concentration

261) *The proportion of body weight represented by total body water content in an extremely obese animal is:*

   a) about 60%
   b) greater than 60%
   c) as much as 75%
   d) as low as 40%

262) *Blood in the canine ejaculate may be associated with any of the following EXCEPT:*

   a) prostatitis
   b) seminal vasculitis
   c) orchitis
   d) ruptured blood vessel on the surface of the penis

263) *Semen is most often collected from dogs by:*

   a) electroejaculation
   b) rectal massage
   c) penile massage
   d) prostatic stimulation

264) *In transvaginal artificial insemination in the bitch, using fresh semen, it should be deposited into the:*

a) uterus
b) vestibule
c) cervical body
d) cranial vagina

265) *An initial rise in plasma progesterone levels in a bitch indicates that:*

a) ovulation has occurred and it is too late to breed the bitch
b) ovulation is imminent and the bitch should be mated in the next few days
c) the bitch is pregnant
d) the bitch is due to whelp within 3 days

266) *In most bitches, the entire oestrous cycle spans:*

a) 4–7 months
b) 21 days
c) 7 days
d) 28 days

267) *In dogs, gestation lasts approximately:*

a) 21 days
b) 30 days
c) 63 days
d) 90 days

268) *In a vaginal smear of a bitch in oestrus, what is the predominant epithelial cell type?*

a) Parabasal cell
b) Non-cornified small intermediate and superficial cell
c) Cornified, large intermediate and superficial cell
d) Red blood cell

269) *Which ONE of the following is NOT an indication for caesarean section in a queen?*

a) Period of more than 4 hours since delivery of the previous kitten
b) Foul smelling, haemorrhagic vulvar discharge
c) Constant straining to deliver kitten
d) Non-odoriferous, brownish vulvar discharge after delivery of the second kitten

270) *Concerning reproduction in cats, which statement is LEAST accurate?*

a) In the Northern Hemisphere, cats are polyestrous from late January to fall
b) In a non-pregnant cat, the corpus luteum produces progesterone for 10 days between heats
c) Cats that have been bred but that are not pregnant may develop pseudopregnancy and show signs of pregnancy
d) Cats that have been bred but that are not pregnant cease cycling for several months

271) *In cats, classic signs of oestrus include all of the following with the EXCEPTION of:*

a) vocalisation, rear-leg treading
b) mounting of the male by the female
c) rubbing and rolling
d) elevated hindquarters (lordosis), tail deflected

272) *In cats, NORMAL signs of copulation, but not necessarily conception, include all of the following with the EXCEPTION of:*

a) the male biting queen's neck while holding the queen between his front legs
b) the queen rolling and licking her vulva in a frenzied manner
c) the queen rejecting the tom for 20–60 minutes
d) draining of white blood-flecked mucus from the queen's vulva

273) *In queens, pregnancy lasts approximately:*

a) 21 days
b) 65 days
c) 90 days
d) 120 days

274) *The function of the lens is to:*

a) transmit visual impulses to the brain
b) enable light rays to focus on the retina
c) provide nourishment to the eye
d) dilate and contrast according to the light intensity

275) *Which ONE of the following hormones is secreted by the posterior pituitary gland?*

   a) Prolactin
   b) Adrenocorticotrophic hormone
   c) Anti-diuretic hormone
   d) Luteinising hormone

276) *Which ONE of the following hormones is secreted by the medulla of the adrenal gland?*

   a) Noradrenaline
   b) Cortisol
   c) Androgens
   d) Aldosterone

277) *Which ONE of the following hormones is not produced by an endocrine gland?*

   a) Chorionic gonadotrophin
   b) Insulin
   c) Somatostatin
   d) Adrenaline

278) *Which ONE of the following is not a function of parathyroid hormone?*

   a) To stimulate osteoclast activity
   b) To inhibit osteoblast activity
   c) To increase the urinary excretion of calcium ions
   d) To stimulate the secretion of calcitriol

279) *Which ONE of the following is an example of a steroid hormone?*

   a) Thyroxin
   b) Follicle-stimulating hormone
   c) Adrenaline
   d) Cortisol

280) *Which ONE of the following hormones is NOT secreted by the pancreas?*

   a) Insulin
   b) Glucagon
   c) Somatostatin
   d) Calcitriol

281) *Which of the following is the layer in the epidermis of the integument where the cells are completely keratinised?*

   a) Stratum granulosum
   b) Stratum corneum
   c) Stratum lucidem
   d) Stratum germinativum

282) *Which layer of skin contains the hair follicles, sweat and sebaceous glands?*

   a) Dermis
   b) Hypodermis
   c) Epidermis
   d) Stratum germinativum

283)   *Where are MOST vibrissae located?*

   a) On the tail of the animal
   b) On the head of the animal
   c) On the foot pads of the animal
   d) On the lateral surfaces of the body of the animal

284)   *Which ONE of the following is NOT a function of the sebaceous glands?*

   a) To secrete sebum
   b) To allow temperature control
   c) To produce pheromones
   d) To waterproof the hair

285)   *Which ONE of the following statements is INCORRECT?*

   a) Mammary glands are modified sweat glands
   b) Anal glands are modified sebaceous glands
   c) Ceruminous glands are modified sweat glands
   d) Meibomian glands are modified sweat glands

286)   *Which layer of skin is formed from stratified squamous epithelial cells?*

   a) Epidermis
   b) Dermis
   c) Hypodermis
   d) All of the above

287) *Which hair type forms the undercoat of an animal?*

a) Vibrissae
b) Wool hair
c) Guard hair
d) Shedding hair

288) *What volume of urine is passed by the average dog per day?*

a) 20 ml/kg body weight
b) 50 ml/kg body weight
c) 10 ml/kg body weight
d) 30 ml/kg body weight

289) *What is the normal pH of urine in the dog?*

a) 3
b) 6
c) 8
d) 8.5

290) *Which ONE of the following is NOT a function of the kidneys in the dog?*

a) Production of renin
b) Excretion of water and waste materials from the body
c) Production of erythropoietin
d) Conversion of ammonia to urea and uric acid

291) *The epiglottis is composed of:*

   a) elastic cartilage
   b) hyaline cartilage
   c) spongy bone
   d) smooth muscle

292) *Which ONE of the following statements is CORRECT?*

   a) The trachea is lined with ciliated epithelium
   b) The trachea is strengthened by incomplete c-shaped rings of fibrocartilage
   c) The trachea is formed from striated muscle
   d) All of the above statements are correct

293) *What is the term given to the exchange of gases across the walls of the alveoli?*

   a) Partial pressure
   b) Osmosis
   c) Diffusion
   d) Filtration

294) *Which ONE of the following statements is INCORRECT? During inspiration:*

   a) the muscles of the diaphragm relax
   b) the external intercostal muscles contract
   c) intrathoracic pressure is decreased
   d) the volume of the thoracic cavity increases

295) *What is the term given to the amount of air breathed in and out during normal respiration?*

    a) Residual volume
    b) Inspiratory capacity
    c) Lung capacity
    d) Tidal volume

296) *Where are the chemoreceptors located that are stimulated by a fall in oxygen content of the blood?*

    a) Medulla oblongata
    b) Lining of the lungs
    c) Aortic arch
    d) All of the above

297) *What increases the transmission of nervous impulses by a neuron?*

    a) Increase in length of the neuron
    b) Myelination
    c) Presence of nodes of Ranvier
    d) Absence of Schwann cells

298) *Which ONE of the following areas is located in the hind brain?*

    a) Thalamus
    b) Hypothalamus
    c) Cerebrum
    d) Pons

299) *From which area could you collect a sample of cerebrospinal fluid?*

   a) Dura mater
   b) Arachnoid mater
   c) Pia mater
   d) Subarachnoid

300) *Which one of the cranial nerves carries impulses associated with sight?*

   a) I
   b) II
   c) V
   d) VIII

Answers

1)	b	23)	a	45)	a	67)	b
2)	b	24)	b	46)	a	68)	d
3)	c	25)	b	47)	b	69)	a
4)	b	26)	c	48)	d	70)	d
5)	d	27)	c	49)	a	71)	c
6)	a	28)	c	50)	c	72)	b
7)	c	29)	b	51)	d	73)	a
8)	c	30)	a	52)	a	74)	c
9)	d	31)	a	53)	a	75)	d
10)	b	32)	c	54)	d	76)	a
11)	d	33)	a	55)	b	77)	d
12)	d	34)	d	56)	c	78)	b
13)	b	35)	a	57)	b	79)	d
14)	a	36)	d	58)	d	80)	b
15)	d	37)	b	59)	c	81)	b
16)	b	38)	d	60)	a	82)	b
17)	d	39)	c	61)	c	83)	c
18)	c	40)	a	62)	c	84)	b
19)	a	41)	d	63)	d	85)	b
20)	a	42)	a	64)	a	86)	d
21)	a	43)	b	65)	b	87)	a
22)	d	44)	c	66)	c	88)	a

89)	b	125)	a	161)	a	197)	b
90)	a	126)	d	162)	c	198)	d
91)	b	127)	d	163)	b	199)	b
92)	b	128)	c	164)	c	200)	c
93)	c	129)	d	165)	d	201)	a
94)	a	130)	d	166)	c	202)	b
95)	d	131)	b	167)	d	203)	d
96)	a	132)	b	168)	a	204)	c
97)	b	133)	c	169)	d	205)	d
98)	b	134)	d	170)	c	206)	b
99)	c	135)	a	171)	c	207)	a
100)	b	136)	d	172)	d	208)	a
101)	d	137)	b	173)	a	209)	b
102)	d	138)	a	174)	b	210)	a
103)	d	139)	b	175)	d	211)	c
104)	b	140)	d	176)	c	212)	a
105)	a	141)	d	177)	d	213)	b
106)	d	142)	c	178)	b	214)	c
107)	b	143)	d	179)	a	215)	b
108)	d	144)	d	180)	c	216)	b
109)	b	145)	b	181)	a	217)	c
110)	d	146)	a	182)	b	218)	a
111)	b	147)	d	183)	c	219)	c
112)	c	148)	c	184)	a	220)	a
113)	a	149)	b	185)	a	221)	c
114)	c	150)	a	186)	b	222)	d
115)	d	151)	c	187)	a	223)	a
116)	b	152)	d	188)	c	224)	b
117)	a	153)	c	189)	d	225)	b
118)	d	154)	a	190)	a	226)	d
119)	d	155)	c	191)	a	227)	a
120)	d	156)	d	192)	a	228)	c
121)	b	157)	c	193)	d	229)	d
122)	b	158)	a	194)	b	230)	c
123)	d	159)	d	195)	d	231)	c
124)	c	160)	c	196)	c	232)	b

233)	c	250)	c	267)	c	284)	b
234)	b	251)	a	268)	c	285)	d
235)	c	252)	c	269)	d	286)	a
236)	c	253)	b	270)	d	287)	b
237)	b	254)	b	271)	b	288)	a
238)	c	255)	b	272)	d	289)	b
239)	c	256)	a	273)	b	290)	d
240)	b	257)	a	274)	b	291)	a
241)	a	258)	a	275)	c	292)	a
242)	c	259)	b	276)	a	293)	c
243)	d	260)	d	277)	a	294)	a
244)	d	261)	d	278)	c	295)	d
245)	c	262)	d	279)	d	296)	c
246)	a	263)	c	280)	d	297)	b
247)	d	264)	d	281)	b	298)	d
248)	d	265)	b	282)	a	299)	d
249)	b	266)	a	283)	b	300)	b

Printed and bound by CPI Group (UK) Ltd, Croydon, CR0 4YY

03/10/2024

01040848-0005